The Cocktail

That is what cured my colon cancer

Lorna Richardson

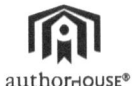
authorHOUSE®

A

Nurse's

Story

AuthorHouse™
1663 Liberty Drive
Bloomington, IN 47403
www.authorhouse.com
Phone: 1-800-839-8640

First published by AuthorHouse   3/22/2011

ISBNP: 978-1-4567-3657-6 (sc)
ISBN: 978-1-4567-3658-3 (hc)

Library of Congress Control Number: 2011902559

Printed in the United States of America

This book is dedicated with great appreciation and love to my mother, Adelaide Marshall.

Contents

Foreword

Faith is a powerful force that propels individuals on their journey to realize restoration. Lorna, in her book, demonstrates the power of faith, strength and courage. A person who remained focused on God's promises and never doubted God's gift - the miraculous Sour Sop tea.

Aimed primarily at the people who are diagnosed with cancer, this book also appeals to all who are facing challenges.

Personally, I think it is a must read.

Karlene Richardson
Licensed Practical Nurse

Acknowledgments

At the completion of my assignment I usually reflect on the people who helped me along the way.

This time how-ever, the list begins with a God I cannot see. He is awesome. He is my Savior and my Friend. Without Him this project would not have been born with such ease, with such love and with such joy.

I am extremely grateful to Karl, my husband, who has been a silent force in my life. I love and appreciate you.

Adelaide Marshall, my dear mother, I thank you for your guidance.

Karlene, my daughter, Gary my son, Tia, Teddy, Lexcy, Lenae, Jada, my grand children, you make me very happy. I am so grateful for all of you.

Clover, Harry, Avis, Carl, Eileen, Marilyn, Grace, Nathan, Nov, Rose, Orville, Claire, Flozel, Milton, Kaye, Sonia, Vava, Betty, Ken, Grace, Sammy, Dorette, Aunt Marjorie, Pat, Huldah, your daily pampering touched the core of my soul.

To my extended family, Pastor Webb and his wife Ethlyn and family Faithlyn, Kayonne, Suzette, Maxine. Thank you for being there for me.

To all my co-workers, especially those in administration, Thank you for being so considerate.

To all my friends, Thank you for demonstrating such love and tenderness.

Words cannot express my gratitude to the oncology team who so kindly and compassionately shared its remarkable world with me.

To the staff of AuthorHouse Publishing Company, Thank you for treating my work with such care and understanding.

In this wake up call to manage her cross, my mother, Lorna Richardson, shares her story - The Cocktail. It is a spiritual stimulant for the soul.

Lorna helps her readers cope with the emotional stress associated with a cancer diagnosis.

She also shows how spiritual transition and the use of the Sour Sop tea were the silent force in her restoration.

Gary Richardson

This book is written with you in mind. You may be the person looking in from the outside or you may be the wounded.

I pray that it will help you cope with the emotional stress associated with challenging experiences.

Spiritual Transition - that is adjusting your thinking, exercising faith and believing God's word is the path to your restoration.

I also hope that the large print has brought you comfortable and pleasurable reading.

Accept Your Cross

Faith never knows where it is being led, but it knows and Loves the one who is leading.

—Oswald Chambers

"I have some bad news for you. You have colon cancer," my doctor calmly said in a matter-of-fact tone. He was looking straight into my eyes as I examined his face. His gaze traveled past my rational mind down to the pit of my stomach then slowly grew into a tightness that gripped my heart. Time simply stopped everywhere in the universe because images flashed through my mind at the speed of thought. The first images were of my patients who I had cared for in the last forty years as a nurse and remembering all the ones who suffered from cancer. My cancer patients were all dead. I could feel my heart constrict and miss a beat.

Obviously, I did not drink enough water, or maybe did not eat enough roughage, and I could have certainly taken better care of myself. Cancer only strikes those who do not live a healthy life--what am I thinking? I am a trained professional and here I am beating my self for getting cancer when I knew that we do not really know what causes cancer.

What is cancer? Cancer is a malignant (progressive and uncontrolled growth) tumor (mass of tissue that serves no purpose). It begins when cells in the body start to grow out of control. Could cancer be the result of a stressful experience? Could it be from some irritant that is picked up along the way? Could cancer develop from a bug I picked up? Any of these possibilities are known to us health professionals, but now it is inside me. What do I do next?

After what seemed like hours passing, the doctor began to speak again. "Are you alright? We need to schedule chemo." I was surprised that the doctor was still in the room. He was a good practitioner. I did not know him personally, but I heard he was knowledgeable and skilled. I decided instantly that I would follow his advice.

He referred me to a chemo doctor - a very pleasant young man who discussed the treatment plan with me. Chemotherapy 24 hours per day, 7 days per week for 6 weeks via a pump. I was also introduced to the chemo nurse who mentioned the possible side effects of the drug - hair loss, weight loss, low blood cell count, nausea and vomiting. The next appointment was with my radiation therapy doctor who scheduled treatment 5 days per week for 6 weeks, starting the same day as the chemo treatment.

The day was almost over. I drove home, but I didn't remember driving. The only thing I remembered was the tightness in my heart. Once home, I sat down in my comfortable chair and began thanking and praising God for protecting me from such a diagnosis for all these years. It seems as though we are protected for a time by an invisible mesh. A mesh that shields us from accident, sickness and death. We walk through this mesh every day, but unaware of its presence. Like the immune system which protects the body from harmful bacteria, so does this invisible mystical mesh protect us from life's threatening situations and challenges.

During this period, life is beautiful, health is great and the years keep rolling along until one day it happens. Without warning the mesh breaks and a picture of a tumor is staring you in the face.

With such a diagnosis as colon cancer - the second deadliest form of cancer - the silent killer, it is easy for one to get bent out of shape and remain disfigured.

This type of challenge requires a resolute, unshakeable faith in God.

In addition to having faith, I know I need to have the willingness to learn how to manage what I just received - my cross.

The question is how am I going to deal with this cross. Am I going to drift into a state of denial? Am I going to waiver in disbelief or break and run?

Whining and self-pity, as logical as they seem, might be harmful so I have to rule those out.

Before going to bed, I decided to pray. But, how do I begin? What do I say to God Almighty now that cancer has invaded my body? Was it my fault? Lord, where do I begin? After feeling sorrow for myself I closed my eyes and cleared my mind.

Oh Lord, Thank you for my life experience. You

have shown me the wonders of your creation. Only you can give us that wonderful and precious breath of life.

Today Oh Lord , I tremble before you because you have decided that my end is near.

My heart is sad because the disease I feared most

is up against me. I feel crippled, like a lame sparrow sitting alone upon a house top.

As I sit Oh Lord, purge me and wash me I pray. Create in me a clean heart and renew a right spirit within me.

Teach me Oh God to do thy will for you are my God. Lead me in the path of righteousness I pray. Take my hand Oh Lord and guide me along the way. Give me wisdom and power so that my last days will be a light, bringing hope to my patients and guiding them through the night.

Thank You for your salvation. It all make sense

Now. YOUR WILL BE DONE. AMEN.

I might have dozed off, but I sat up because I heard a sweet soft voice in the background.

"Lorna Delle your diagnosis is not a mistake. It is your cross that has a sacred purpose and will be used for your good. So do not fear, for I am with you. Do not be dismayed, for I am your God. I will strengthen you and help you. I will uphold you with My righteous right hand.

The next day I went to work feeling peaceful. The day went quickly. My patients seem different. These were wonderful people-I understood how they felt. I could feel every emotion they felt. I understood my patients were sick and needed someone to know what pain they felt deep inside their souls. I love my patients. It is funny how tragedy changes one's image of fellow humans. We are all such precise creatures-God's creatures.

That evening I called my pastor, Jeffery Webb. A Jamaican, he is very spiritual and glowed with God's love. I asked him to pray for me for I have colon cancer. I expected Reverend Webb to pour compassion and sympathy over the phone, but instead he began to tell me about a cure for cancer. Being a little skeptical, I let him finish speaking without listening to his "miracle cure" story-these stories are entirely myths and as a professional health provider, I do not believe in them. Pastor Webb promised to meet with me after Sunday service. So I thanked him and hung up.

His sermon was exceptional that Sunday. I felt warm with the love of Jesus, my Lord and Savior. Pastor Webb came up to me after service and took me to his backyard where a very pretty tree grew. "I planted this sour Sop tree fifteen years ago when I first emigrated from Jamaica." "Oh, that's nice" I said, thinking he is very nice to make small talk before letting me bleed my pain on his shoulder. "Lorna, my mother had cancer." Pointing to the tree he said, "The doctors said that they could do nothing for her-that was 32 years ago and she is still healthy because of the Sour Sop tree and prayer."

I watched his composure, but he did not show any deceit or showmanship. "Are you saying this tree cures cancer?" I demanded-instantly regretting my harsh tone of voice. "My wife's sister had lung cancer and was assigned to Hospice." He stated with conviction, "I don't know if she is cured, but while in Hospice, she gained weight, is very energetic, and looks great." "Let me give you some to drink." and began clipping without waiting for me to speak. "Take one leaf, a piece of branch, and boil them for one minute in a cup of water. Drink a cup without sugar everyday for three months.

I have never before felt annoyed and curious at the same time. What do I do? I decided politeness is the better behavior to show my pastor and accepted the foliage. I left without the sympathy I expected to receive. Driving home, I calmed down and began to accept the fact that God works in mysterious ways. So I started making my Sour Sop tea and planning on drinking a cup without sugar every day.

After drinking my first cup of tea, I remembered a dream I had three months earlier – An elderly woman gave me a Sour Sop fruit. What does this really mean? I was completely overwhelmed. My body started to vibrate. It was almost too much for me to take in.

I arrived at my first chemotherapy treatment on time. After being escorted to the chemo suite, I sat down in a very comfortable chair. My treatment lasted only 15 minutes. My blood was tested. The nurse prepared the medication in a plastic bag which was then placed in a small case. Because the chemo medication is given intravenously, I had a PICC (peripherally inserted central catheter) inserted in my right upper arm and advanced all the way to my heart. This procedure was done two days earlier. The chemo medication was attached to my PICC line and then the pump was turned on. The nurse was very pleasant-we chatted quite a lot as two professionals-but never about cancer. Now it's time for me to see the doctor. I was escorted to the examining room. I remember the day rectal bleeding occurred which seemed like only yesterday. The flow was enough to warn me that I should see a physician. I also felt chest pain, but I did not believe it was related until my blood work was done-low hemoglobin was the result. The doctor felt a rectal mass and ordered a colonoscopy. The test result brought him to the diagnosis colon cancer. A CAT scan confirmed the diagnosis. Now my symptoms were getting worse. I felt weak, blood was showing in my abnormal appearing stools. My hemoglobin went down to 10.1 where the normal level should have been 11-14.

My doctor entered the room. With a strange look on his face he said, "Lorna, removal of the tumor by a surgeon will be necessary.

This will be followed by another round of chemotherapy. And don't be surprised if you have to get a colostomy." This is an opening of part of the colon onto the abdominal wall which serves as an exit site for feces-in other words it is an artificial anus.

I was speechless, I felt like crying, but I thought shedding tears in certain places, especially the doctor's office, might be misconstrued-psychotic behavior? Depression? Who knows.

I felt like crying for patients who are struggling to manage their colostomies. I felt like crying. The tears took over my entire eyes clouding my vision. I felt like crying, but I didn't want the other nurses to think that I am weak, angry, sad or frightened.

I am now alone in the examining room. Alone with my thoughts and feelings. I really want to cry, but instead of crying I moved the muscles of my upper lip northward. I did it so skillfully, the tears that originated in the upper corner of my eyes found their way to the opposite end. Now I can go home and no one would know that I really wanted to cry.

There was a rap on the door. A nurse brought me my appointment card which I could not read. Tears flooded my eyes, but I never lost a drop.

Although I lack eloquence in speech, I feel compelled to tell my story. How could I not show appreciation to a God who from His garden picked, bagged and delivered my healing medication. A God who spared me all the side effects of chemotherapy and radiation therapy.

How could I not love a God who heard my cry and moved into action. Like a roaring lion He acted as my attorney. He stood between the surgeon and myself and said. "No one dare tamper with my child. How can you remove a tumor you cannot see? How can you remove a tumor you cannot feel? How can you remove a tumor without knowing its location?" A God who reached down and tenderly removed me from my surgeon's grip. Why shouldn't I wash His feet with my tears? A God who provided the last ingredient for my cancer cure cocktail and defended me for His glory and for my good. Why shouldn't I?

2

The Gift

God works in mysterious ways, and this is one of the most mysterious gifts ever given to me--a tree.

Considering most modern medicines come from organic extracts found in nature--extracts that have not even scratched down a fraction to the total depth of all that God created--I was compelled to research what this tree had that could compel people to make such miraculous claims.

The internet made even more miraculous claims to even cite respectable science research--is this true? Articles quoted respected research institutions, but to weed through internet nonsense, the best policy is to go straight to the actual written research report. The doctors or hospital who conducted the research as well as the publication that published it come to question.

Much to my surprise, Graviola (species *Annona Muricata*) commonly called Sour Sop, Brazilian Paw Paw, and many other herbal names boasted resepectable science. In 1976, the National

Cancer Institute found the leaves and stem of Sour Sop tree showed active cytotoxicity (toxic to living cells) against cancer cells.

Three other research groups have isolated compounds in the seeds and leaves of Sour Sop that demonstrated anti-tumorous and selective toxicity against various types of cancer cells. They published eight clinical studies. One study from the Catholic University of South Korea demonstrated that Sour Sop was selectively catatonic to colon cancer cells and was 10,000 times the potency of chemotherapy, Adriamycin (a commonly used chemotherapy drug). The study went on to say Sour Sop effectively targeted malignant cells while leaving healthy cells untouched.

In 1998, four new studies narrowed down specific phytochemicals (a chemical substance obtained from plants that is biologically active, but not nutritious) that demonstrate the strongest anticancerous and antiviral properties. A study from Purdue University showed that this chemical from the Sour Sop killed cancer cells and were especially effective against prostate, pancreatic, and lung cancers.

Cancer research is ongoing on Sour Sop. Considering the huge cost to conduct research, companies like to invest in something that has potential benefits and do not fund research on myths--Ok, I am now impressed. Let me try this gift from God.

I examined the leaves and bark closer--beautiful leaves, strong "barky" odor, and definite herbal flavor--it seemed like ordinary plant material. After giving thanks to Jesus, I prepared a brew--it tasted slightly like bark mostly from smell, slightly caustic, but the flavor was not too bad. I drank a cup every evening as Jeffrey had said to do. After a week, I began to flavor the tea. A fruit drink is made by blending the pulp from the fruit in water and adding condensed milk with cinnamon, nutmeg and a dash of rum, producing a nectar-like consistency. Three weeks drinking Sour Sop tea reduced my symptoms--rectal bleeding, general weakness and low hemoglobin.

Graviola is a small, upright evergreen tree growing ten feet in height with large dark green and glossy leaves. It is indigenous to most of the warmest tropical areas in South and North America, including the Amazon. It produces a large heart-shaped edible fruit that is 6--9 inches, yellow-green in color, with white flesh. The fruit is sold in local markets in the tropics where it is called Guanabana or Brazilian Cherimoya. All parts of the Graviola tree are used in natural medicine in the tropics including the bark, leaves, roots, fruit and fruit seeds. Different properties and uses are attributed to the different parts of the tree. Generally, the fruit and fruit juice are taken for worms and parasites, to cool fevers, to increase mother's milk after childbirth, and as an astringent for diarrhea and dysentery. The crushed seeds are used as a vermifuge (a medication capable of causing the evacuation of parasitic intestinal worms) and anathematic (capable of expelling or destroying parasitic worms) against internal and external parasites and worms. The bark, leaves and roots are considered a sedative, antispasmodic (a drug used to relieve or prevent spasms), hypertensive (having abnormally high blood pressure) and nervine (having the quality of acting upon or affecting the nerves; quieting nervous excitement) and a tea is made for various disorders for those purposes.

Graviola has a long rich history of use in herbal medicine, as well as, a long recorded indigenous use. In the Peruvian Andes, a leaf tea is used for catarrh (inflammation of the nose and throat with increased production of nucus) and the crushed seed is used to kill parasites. In the Peruvian Amazon, the bark, roots and leaves are used for diabetes and as a sedative and antispasmodic. Indigenous tribes in Guyana use a leaf and/or bark tea of Graviola as a sedative and heart tonic. In the Brazilian Amazon, a leaf tea is used for liver problems and the oil of the leaves and unripe fruit is mixed with olive oil and used externally for neuralgia (acute spasmodic pain along the course of one or more nerves), rheumatism and arthritis pain. In Jamaica, Haiti and the West Indies, the fruit and/or fruit juice is used for fevers, parasites, as a lactagogue (ability to increase quantity of nursing milk) and diarrhea, and the bark or leaves are used as an antispasmodic, sedative, and nervine for heart conditions, coughs, grippe (an acute and highly contagious viral disease causing a high body fever), difficult childbirth, asthma, asthenia (an abnormal loss of strength), hypertension and parasites.

In the June issue of Cancer Letters, Purdue researchers

reported that an isolated compound, *hullatacin,* found in Graviola preferentially killed multi-drug resistant cancer cells because it blocked production of adenosine triphosphate (or ATP, the chief energy-carrying compound in the body). In 1997, Purdue University published information with promising news that several compounds are not only effective in killing tumors that have proven resistant to anti-cancer agents, but also seem to have a special affinity for such resistant cells.

Cancer cells that survive chemotherapy may develop resistance to the agent originally used against them, as well as, to other unrelated drugs. The term multi-drug resistance (MDR) has been applied to this phenomenon. Cancer research will obviously be Ongoing on this important plant and plant chemicals as several pharmaceutical companies continue to research, test and attempt to synthesize these chemicals into new chemotherapeutic (of or relating to chemotherapy) drugs.

Graviola is safe enough that it protects healthy cells instead of killing them, doesn't cause extreme nausea or hair loss and this treatment doesn't make cancer patients drop huge amounts of weight, get weak, or compromise their immune systems.*

Sitting comfortably in my home office, wearing a light robe, I decided to continue with my investigation of this miraculous plant--the Sour Sop tree.

I made several calls, mostly to my friends in Jamaica, WI, pausing only to take sips of the Sour Sop tea which I made early that morning.

It has a very strange taste and an unusual smell, but nevertheless I continued to sip.

"Tell me more," I said. I was listening to a story about Yvonne, a nurse who had cancer and a husband who helped her regain her health. Yvonne, who was diagnosed with cancer of the lymph nodes, had pain in her limbs, abdomen and groin, spasms in her legs and night sweats. She had chemotherapy, but after a while the symptoms came back. A CT scan and PET scan were done and both were conclusive. Cancer was indeed invading Yvonne's lymph nodes once again.

The story continues. When Yvonne started having restless nights and cold sweats, her husband feared the worst. He continued to pray and advised Yvonne to try the Sour Sop tea. After a month, Yvonne had no more pain and went to her doctor for a check-up. Her baffled doctor told them that the cancer movement had stopped. "Joy, unspeakable joy, was what the love birds felt."

For me, things took a very interesting and positive twist.

After three weeks of prayer, praise and pampering, three weeks of chemotherapy and radiation therapy, three weeks of my daily cup of Sour Sop tea, all the signs and symptoms of the disease--what I could see and feel--disappeared. I feel healthy, extremely energetic. My CBC results got better, I gained weight.

Three weeks later the repeat CT scan report failed to mention anything about a malignant tumor that once existed.

Now the Sour Sop tea has dominated my thoughts every waking minute and my dreams every night.

Secretly, I began making plans to share my gift with everyone I knew with a cancer diagnosis. This has to be a secret. After all, I am a professional. What defense would I have if side effects resulted from such a treatment?

Convinced of the rightness of my plan, I considered ways to share my gift.

A quick call to Maxine and then a visit to her home. There I saw her mother lying on the floor. She has been suffering from lung cancer for sometime. I shared the information I received pertaining to the Sour Sop tea and told her that it might make her feel a little better.

I emphasized, "I cannot say it will cure your cancer, but it might make you feel a little better." I shared my gift with her and left.

My return visit was a month later. I was invited to her birthday party. I was literally blown away. I was amazed. This woman was dancing. She gained weight. She looked great.

This situation defines nursing. It's scary, it's heartbreaking, frustrating, dirty, dangerous but, oh my God, absolutely rewarding.

Early one morning, on my way home from work, a co-worker

stopped me in the hallway. "Lorna", she said, "I don't have cancer, but I sure don't want to get it. Could I have some of those leaves?" Instantly, I was transported back to the hills of Ritchies from whence I came. Several fruit trees were on that 10 acre farm. But, was there a Sour Sop tree? Could the farm now accommodate Sour Sop Trees? My supply is running out.

If my offering a cup of Sour Sop tea, seen or unseen, makes a person feel better for a day, a month, six months or a year, then I believe I am accomplishing God's will.

When faced with a stressful situation, God may seem silent, remote or even imaginary. You now see your problem as a real big one. You need something tangible, something that will relieve anxiety without knocking you out. You need relief.

If the Sour Sop tea is the answer, why not? If it will spare you the horrible side effects of chemo and relieve you of the symptoms associated with your disease, why shouldn't you share a cup with me?

God uses the dark periods of our lives to show us the power of His love and to draw us closer to Him.

Our job is to let go, trust Him and be willing to move. Someone once said, "You cannot steer a car that isn't moving."

I have made the choice to move. Now I can hear that same sweet voice saying:

"Lorna Delle, I need you to be my vessel of mercy and compassion. I need a nurse whose compassion is rooted in memories of a scary diagnosis.

Your nursing experience is a gift you can share. You can be of great help to those who are struggling with what you have survived.

I want you to share your gift with the young and the old, the rich and the poor. I am a God of everyone."

Is there a Divine Purpose behind all this?

If you are willing to embrace that possibility, then there might be light at the end of every cancer diagnosis.

3

Love From The Heart

. . .The God of love and peace shall be with you.

2 Corinthians 13:11

When a good friend prays for you during your challenging periods, when you receive cards and letters saying, "I love you," when you receive a hug at a time when you really needed it, it is God's way of letting you know that He is near.

The door bell rang. I peeped through the window. There was my church sister who I love dearly. I opened the door and said, "please come in." "Not yet, I have to go back to my car," she replied. Sister went back to her car three times for three pots with beef soup, chicken soup and peas soup. Three large pots. I greeted her with a hug and then dashed for my room.

I knelt at the side of my bed - a place reserved for special communication with God. I looked up at the ceiling and said, "God tell me, is this my last meal on earth? What am I going to do with so much soup?" Later that evening my pastor, his wife and my son visited. I was so happy, I set the table with the best of everything and proudly stated, "you have choices - chicken soup, beef soup, peas soup - enjoy!"

I went back to my favorite spot in my bedroom and said, "God, thank you. I didn't have to waste any of the soup."

The next day my cell phone rang. I looked at it and there was a call coming in from my job. "Good morning, this is Lorna," I said. The voice said, "yesterday I cried so much. Today I am crying even more." I recognized the voice and then asked "Why are you crying?" "I am going to miss you", she replied. "Where am I going? I asked. "Please don't get me crying again" she replied. My co-worker invited me to church. It was a spirit filled day.

I heard a story not too long ago about a church brother who was driving his truck along a narrow mountain road. As he was negotiating a curve he lost control of the vehicle. It plunged several feet over the side of the mountain. He prayed and was miraculously ejected before the truck burst into flames. God provided a bush that he nervously held onto with his feet dangling. After trying to pull himself up for several minutes, he shouted, "God where are you?" In a few seconds the thundering voice of the Lord echoed back, "I am here, what do you want?" "Please save me. I cannot hold on much longer." The voice replied, "I am your God. I will save you, but first you must release your grip. I am waiting to catch you." The man looked around. Beneath him was his burning truck. Then he shouted, "Lord you've got to be kidding."

My church sisters and brothers have not yet used the word cancer when talking to me. That word apparently is not in their vocabulary or they are simply saying, "God you've got to be kidding."

I couldn't wait to reach my room, that special area in my room. An area that seems to bring comfort and peace. While on my knees, I lifted up my hands and said, "Oh my God I need you. I cannot go through this alone. Lord I cannot hold on any longer. I am willing to let go of my grip so that you can catch me." Within seconds I could hear the same familiar voice. "Lorna Delle, your diagnosis is not a mistake. It was preordained. It is your cross that has a sacred purpose and will be used for your good. So do not fear for I am with you. Do not be dismayed for I am your God. I will strengthen you and help you. I will uphold you with my righteous right hand."

I jumped up and started skipping and singing. There was no

melody, but I was singing anyway. "This is my cross and I will courageously pick it up and follow my Lord, my Savior and friend. He has promised to take this hardship and bring good from it and I believe every word, even if it cost me my life."

The phone rang. My mother said, "Delle, don't worry, we are praying for you." The phone rang again. My sister, brothers, brother-in-law, other relatives, friends, acquaintances called with the same message. We are praying for you. My church sisters and brothers, who refused to use the word "cancer" in our previous conversations, visited and we had a wonderful service together.

My daughter had a different message. "Mommy, I am a nurse. I will be your caregiver." My son said that he went to a nearby church and prayed until he fell asleep. When he woke up everything was so peaceful. He knows that I will be healed.

My mother, sister, brother-in-law and friends felt the same way too.

My husband, who stood by me day in and day out, took me to all my doctors appointments and to the diagnostic centers. Speaking of diagnostic center, with state-of-the-art equipment, seem to terrorize those they serve. X-ray machines, CT (computed tomography) scan machines, MRI (magnetic resonance imaging) machines are all waiting to greet you.

I looked around the waiting room at the faces of those who were waiting patiently to be served. No smiles were seen. Their nerves seem to be rattling with uncertainty. I took a seat and as I bent my knees my confidence began to crumble. "Lorna Richardson, please come this way." The way led me to my CT scan machine.

This machine, a state-of-the-art equipment, confirmed my large colorectal malignant tumor.

I got home late that evening only to find some beautiful cards from some beautiful people awaiting me. The messages were the same, "we are praying for you," "we love you." There were several messages and jokes via e-mails. I could not trade my family and friends for anything in this world.

Before retiring for the night, I picked up my Bible and said a short prayer.

"Lord, what shall I do?" Then I opened the Bible with the hope of doing some research. The very first sentence that my eyes rested on was Acts 22, verse 10. "And I said what shall I do Lord." My entire body shook like a leaf.

With shaking hands, I turned the pages. Matthew 8:3 tells me that Jesus heals with mercy and compassion. He touched the festering sores of the leper and the crusted lids of blinded eyes. Matthew 9:29.

The sick were brought to Jesus and all who touched His garment were healed. Matthew 14:35, 36.

I continued to turn the pages. Then I stopped at Deuteronomy 4:29, "If you seek Him you will find Him." I need to find Him. Why am I feeling exhausted physically, emotionally and spiritually? Why am I at a complete loss when I know how grateful and happy I am for those beautiful cards, letters, gifts, jokes and all that love and affection that keep pouring in.

What have I done to deserve all this, I ask? Very little and sometimes nothing at all, if I may answer my own question.

I know God will give me the wisdom to discover the true meaning of life and the reason behind all the prayers and pampering I am receiving. Through your pampering I can feel God's gentleness, His kindness and His love. I can see His eagerness to touch me and heal me. I recognize His power and His ability to bring peace in my heart.

I also recognize the need to have a closer relationship with my Lord. If you are like me searching for such a relationship, if you have enjoyed success with all its trappings and still there is a feeling of emptiness inside of you, a feeling of loneliness or a dull ache signaling that something is missing, then you need to meet my Lord, my savior, my healer, my surgeon and my friend. With outstretched hands He is inviting you to believe in Him. To trust Him. He is waiting to hold you, to bless you, to heal you. He is waiting to protect you from any weapon that is formed against you. When you are in His arms there will be no dryness in your spirit and no emptiness in your life.

Having a closer relationship with God takes time and discipline.

Just as a flower needs sunshine, water and food so we need nourishment before we can bloom.

In the process of renewing our minds and getting closer to God we must be determined to believe only what can be measured against His word.

As we close this chapter let us sing this beautiful chorus:

> *"Have thine own way Lord*
> *Have thine own way*
> *Thou art the Potter, I am the clay*
> *Mold me and make me after Thy will*
> *While I am waiting yielded and still"*
>
> —George Stebbins

4

Life Will Test You

My brethren count it all joy when we fall into diverse temptations.
Knoweth this that the trying of your faith worketh patience

James 1:2 & 3

That imaginary mesh, the mystical mesh that has been protecting you all these years is torn. You can now see and feel the storms wind and the rain.

What do these represent? Could it be your cancer diagnosis? Life will test you. Faith never seems to go unchallenged for long.

"Why would God permit this to happen?" is a question many people ask.

To answer this question let's go back to the Bible. The Holy Scripture depicts God as loving and kind, tenderly watching over His earthly children and guiding the steps of the faithful. He speaks of us s the people of His pasture, the flock under His care - Psalm 95:7.

My friend God sees you where you are. He is a God of love and of grace. The Bible says He has great plans for you. "For I know the thoughts that I think towards you. Thoughts of peace and not of evil, to give you an expected end." Jeremiah 29:11

Why me? We need to know that it is ok to be human. We live in a world of unanswered questions. We find ourselves in a tug-of-war between fear and trust. But that does not mean that God has turned His back on us. Nor does it mean that God is obligated to explain Himself nor His purpose for our lives.

God wants you to trust Him and lean on His promises.

Today the psalmist is reminding you to go to the Lord with all your concerns.

"Cast your burden upon the Lord and He shall sustain thee. He shall never suffer the righteous to be moved. Psalm 55:22. Jesus also promises peace. "Peace I leave with you and peace I give unto you. Not as the world giveth give I unto you. Let not your heart be troubled, neither let it be afraid." John 14:27.

In other words, the Lord is saying stop, do not allow yourself to be agitated or disturbed. And do not permit yourself to be fearful, to be a coward and become unsettled because of a cancer diagnosis.

God wants to heal you and restore you so that you will be a blessing to the lives of others.

He wants to use you in a mighty way. It's a reason why you are asked to bear this cross. It is for God's glory and your good. So don't panic. There is good news. You do not have to fight this disease alone. The Lord will never leave you nor forsake you.

He is the refuge for the cancer victim and He promises that He will not give you more than you can bear.

God heals by putting you in touch with experts from the required disciplines: pathology, surgery, medical, oncology, radiation.

Multidisciplinary communication and coordination of care are becoming the norm. Doctors from various specialties are coming together to share their talents and experiences to compose a tailored state-of-the-art treatment plan aimed at the best possible outcome for each patient.

The good news is chemotherapy and radiation therapy are becoming easier to handle because of the wide range of cancer research. Just believe God's word. He has promised that your temptation will not be greater than you can bear.

God also heals in ways that cannot be explained medically. Just continue to pray and believe His word. He will rescue you and give you a second chance. He sends help through many channels.

Who knows, the cancer cure cocktail could be your cure as well.

What causes cancer? According to the Taber's Medical Dictionary, the exact cause of cancer is unknown, and further states that unregulated disorganized proliferation of cell growth may be caused by various forms of chronic irritation.

Cancer is invasive and tends to metastasize to new sites. It spreads directly into surrounding tissue and my also be disseminated through the lymphatic and circulatory systems. Many types of cancer can be effectively treated and cured. Some warning signals are unusual bleeding. A lump or thickening in any area, especially the breast. A sore that does not heal. A change in bowel and bladder habits. Hoarseness or persistent cough or unexplained weight loss.

In colorectal cancer, the most common presenting symptoms are bleeding with defecation. The stool may be streaked or mixed with blood. It may also cause constipation or diarrhea and increased stool frequency. A sensation of incomplete evacuation my be present.

Diagnosis is made by various means. The most important one biopsy of the tumor and CAT Scan - Computerized Axial Tomography.

Again, your doctor will discuss this with you.

Screening is usually done by fecal occult blood testing or colonoscopy. Regular colorectal screening is the most powerful weapon in fighting colon cancer.

Colonoscopy is an examination of the upper portion of the sigmoid colon with an elongated speculum.

The colon is the large intestine from the end of the ileum to the anus. It is about five feet (1.5 meters) long and is divided into the ascending, transverse, descending and the sigmoid colon.

It is important that you discuss future screening and specific treatment plans with your doctor.

As you prepare for your treatment you might become anxious. Chemotherapy can be a bit scary, but try to relax and focus on your healthy future. Millions of people have gone through it and are doing well as a result. By now I imagine you have met your chemo care team. Your medical oncologist, your oncology nurse, your primary care physician and your radiation therapy team as well.

You now have the right to information. Your doctor will discuss treatment options. If you don't understand everything about your condition ask for further explanation. You are a participant in your own care. Get involved. When it comes to communicating with your cancer team there are no dumb questions.

You need to know what type of cancer you have and the location of the tumor. Discuss the possible side effects of the chemo drugs. Ask about the help you should expect if you suffer a serious reaction.

Chemo drugs are powerful agents designed to stop the growth and destroy cancer cells in the body. It is very important that you do not miss an appointment and try to be on time every time.

A calendar with all the appointment written down can be a great help.

I am reminded of a patient who was sitting in the chemo suite of the doctor's office. She greeted everyone as they entered the room. She was so pleasant, I looked at her and said, "I take it your treatment is over or almost over." She looked at me with a smile and said, "I have another year to go." I could not hold back my tears of gratitude. This patient has one year to go and I have six weeks. One year. Could my nerves handle it? I wouldn't be surprised if the nurse thought I was crazy, but I started singing. "One day at a time, sweet Jesus. That's all I'm asking from you."

Please join me:

One day at a time, sweet Jesus. That's all I'm asking from you.

Just give me the strength to do everyday what I have to do.

Yesterday's gone, sweet Jesus, and tomorrow may never be mine.

Lord, help me today. Show me the way. One day at a time.

Your cross might not be a cancer diagnosis. It might be a broken relationship that hurts way down to the core of your soul.

"Oh God, forgive me when I shout and jump on the pulpit. It is not because of the Holy Spirit Lord, It is because of that sister. She has a seductive walk and when she blinks her eyelids I can feel pins and needles throughout my body. That is why I left my wife Lord. My wife is too decent, too clean and when I hold her the pins and needles are not there. Now she is gone, leaving my church sister and me. I thought I had enough reason to celebrate. We cling to each other like a vine to a wall. I squeezed her so tight Lord, when I open my hands she is not there.

Lord, I am jumping and shouting on the pulpit, not because of the Holy Spirit, but because my church sister is now in the arms of another church brother. Lord, this cross is more than I can bear.

Have you seen an abused woman lately? You can't tell from the clothes she wears or her fancy hairstyle. You cannot describe her by race nor by the type of car she drives. But. her pain can be seen through her eyes. The tears that come out at night seem to leave permanent marks on her face. She is sad. She finds herself arguing with people who are not listening. She is in a frightening relationship that is holding her hostage. She seems to be buried down under the weight and pressures that come from deep dark secrets.

It is the uncertainty of this relationship, the uncertainty of the future that forces her to seek a God who can see where her frail eyes can't. A God who can rescue her.

"Oh my God", she cried. "Please save my children. They are smothered by the vulgarity in the home. Exposed to pornography as they grow up in the closet. Peeping and hiding from the acts of cruelty and crime. Lord, touch my children so that they won't have to face what I am facing. Lord, please speak peace to this home and deliverance to this family. Lord, I surrender all."

Although you might have many regrets, although your past my be filled with pain, although you might have made many mistakes, failed and sinned, don't worry God is very comfortable working with broken people.

There are many examples throughout the Holy Scriptures where God restored and used broken people. For example, Moses, Paul and Peter.

When you are experiencing brokenness you don't have to hide

behind a mask. God wants to erase those scars. He wants to cleanse you and use your challenges for His glory and for your good. You are a survivor. Some little boy, some little girl needs to know the recipe for survival. Somewhere in the street there is someone dying because she does not know that it is possible to live through what you have already endured.

Pray with these little boys and girls. Teach them how to trust God and how to praise Him. Pamper them. Love them.

Now we can all sing.

"Amazing Grace, how sweet the sound
That saved a wretch like me.
I once was lost, but now am found.
Was blind, but now I see."

Life will test you. Many foolish men have plunged into a ditch of despair trying to create a jewel from an ordinary stone. Wake up oh ye men, things that come easily generally tarnish quickly. The pursuit of a wife can be very challenging, but the wise man knows that a good wife is a woman waiting to be discovered. She is the missing ingredient that will complete your vision.

Now that you have found this beautiful jewel, this priceless diamond, this wonderful and divine expression of love, you start questioning her motives. You treat her loving deeds with total indifference.

Is there something wrong with you? If so, unconditional love will show you the truth. Examine yourself. Acknowledge your own shortcomings. Look how many times you have begged God for a gentle, spiritual, fun-loving woman to share your life. God sent you a woman who fits the bill and you are now trying to find everything wrong with her.

Life will test you.

The greatest commandment as stated in the Holy Scriptures is the one that commands us to love the Lord with all our heart, soul and mind and the second to love our neighbors as ourselves. But, how can we love our neighbors when we have not learned to love ourselves. Is it possible that this could be the basis for so many dysfunctional relationships? Is it possible that because we see ourselves as insignificant, inferior, with very little or no value, we open ourselves to a life of abuse? Life will test you.

People have a tendency to treat us the way we treat ourselves. People with low self-esteem seem to attract people who dominate, control or belittle them. There are many people who endure abuse. Abuse in many forms because they are afraid of being alone.

You might also find yourself surrounded by negative, cranky, annoying, aggravating, unreasonable cantankerous people. There are some who get "under your skin" and the others "sit on your one last nerve." These are our neighbors. Even if they drive us nuts, we cannot stop loving them. True love - the kind that sent Jesus from Heaven to earth all the way to the Roman Cross. That kind of love wins all the time. This type of love is medicine for the sick. It cures. it cures those who give it and those who receive it.

Such is the power of love. We need to see love, to hear it and to feel it, and to know how to pass it along to others.

When we can truly love our neighbor as ourselves we will have fulfilled the law of God. Leviticus 1:1. In that sense love leads us back to the Golden Rule - "Do unto others as you would have them do unto you. Matthew 7:12.

There is no doubt your faith is shaken. I know you are hurting. I can imagine the pain you are experiencing after you have exercised faith, after you have prayed for healing for yourself and your loved ones and God says "no".

Don't assume that God is silent or his apparent inactivity means that He does not care. You are wrong. He is at work in His own unique way. The psalmist assures us that "the eyes of the Lord are on the righteous and His ears are attentive to their prayers. First Peter 3:12.

The Lord might choose not to grant a request that you think is vitally important. Isaiah 55:89 teaches "For my thoughts are not your thoughts, neither are our ways my ways declares the Lord."

Sometimes we are asked to endure things that cause discomfort and pain. Sometimes we are asked to release our loved ones. Allow him to put down the physical form and lay aside his garment that was meant only for temporary use. Release him as he steps aside into the divine level of spiritual existence.

We will experience a natural loss for awhile because we have grown accustomed to having our loved one here with us physically.

Our loved one has passed. To pass means to move on or ahead or proceed. Our journey here on this earth has the illusion of permanence, but we should not be fooled. We are just passing through.

The death that we see is only the beginning of a new life, the transformation into a new form and, therefore, should not be seen as a tragedy, but a triumph. The apostle Paul puts it this way. "Oh death where is thy string, oh grave where is they victory." 1 Corinthians 15:55.

When God says no to your healing prayers, don't worry He has promised to take these hardships and bring good from them. Romans 8:28 says, "All things work together for good to them that love God, to them who are called according to His purpose."

While you are on earth you may never see the purpose of your suffering, but God's word is true. Peter left no doubt in our minds when he wrote "Behold, think it not strange concerning the fiery trial which is to try you as though some strange thing happened unto you. But rejoice in as much as ye are partakers of Christ's sufferings that when His glory shall be revealed ye may be glad also with exceeding joy. 1 Peter 4:12-13.

Solomon in Ecclesiastes 11:5 states, "As thou knowest not what is the way of the spirit nor how the bones do grow in the womb of her that is with child, even so thou knowest not the works of God who maketh all."

The scriptures tell us that "The secret things belong to the Lord our God" Deuteronomy 29:29, and warns us "Lean not on your own understanding." Proverbs 3:5.

Clearly, unless the Lord chooses to explain Himself to us, His motivation and purpose are beyond our understanding.

If we could fully comprehend how deeply loved we are by our creator, we would never shed a tear when our loved one passes. It is very comforting to know that the very presence of the King of Kings, the creator of Heaven and earth hovers around your loved one. It is also comforting to know that Jesus will arrive at the precise moment necessary to fulfill God's purpose - to escort your loved one to glory.

I am reminded of how confused and sad Jesus' disciples were after their master ws crucified on the Roman cross. As they walked towards the village of Emmaus they shared their thoughts and feelings "as they talked together of all the things which had happened. Jesus Himself drew near and walked with them, but they could not see Him." Luke 24: 14-15.

The Bible also states that the disciples were kept from recognizing Him.

How often do we become so absorbed in our suffering that we fail to recognize God's presence. We fail to hear His message. When a new trial comes our way we become sad. We fail to remember all the good things God did for us in the past. When we cannot pay our bills we fail to remember the amount of bills He paid for us. We grumble when we are faced with a difficult diagnosis or a broken relationship. God knows our weaknesses. He knows we have a tendency to forget what we have already seen Him do. For our good, He draws our attention to our lack of faith, but heals us if we believe, to demonstrate His power. Note what happened to His disciples after His crucifixion. They were confused. They could not imagine that their master allowed Himself to be crucified on the Roman cross. As they walked the dusty road to Emmaus they did not know that they were about to be given the greatest news ever heard by human ears and that they would be given their greatest assignment.

"Go ye therefore and teach all nations, baptizing them in the name of the Father, and of the Son, and of the Holy Ghost. Teaching them to observe all things whatsoever I have commanded you and lo I am with you always even unto the end of the world." Matthew 28:19-20.

If you find your self on that dusty road to Emmaus-sad, confused, depressed-trust God. If your prayers do not bring immediate relief, do not assume they are not heard. It is my firm conviction that the Lord answers every prayer. He might say "no", He might say "yes" or He might say "I will, only if you allow me to."

"For as high as the Heavens are above the earth, so great is His love for those who fear Him." Psalm 103:11. So when God say "no" He still loves us. Someday we will be glad that it was His will and not ours that was done.

5

The Path

In all thy ways acknowledge Him
And He shall direct your path.

Proverbs 3.6

Trust and obey. This is the first step we have to take towards our restoration. Trusting God is a process. it is a step of faith. Trusting God requires obedience.

Sometimes it will appear as though God has forgotten about us, but is not so. When we put our trust in God we can comfortably lean on His promises.

The psalmist puts it this way. "Oh taste and see that the Lord is good. Blessed is the man who trust in Him." Psalm 34:8

As we continue on the path towards our restoration we will realize how important it is to forgive. But, what is forgiveness. Forgiveness means letting go of the anger and the desire for revenge.

When we really let go of the hurt people have caused us God knows and the end result is a change in the way we feel. No longer are we bitter or angry. The memories will keep coming back, but if we let go and refuse to dwell on the problem it will slowly fade away.

Without forgiveness there is no healing.

Without forgiveness there is no recovery.

Without forgiveness there is no future.

Forgiveness, therefore, is a choice, a decision we make to release others fro their sins against us.

When God forgives us of our sins he blots them out and remembers them no more. Hebrews 19:17

There in my bed, I realized how dependent on God I was. Totally dependent. I feel broken, weak and useless. Useless because I feel inadequate. I am no longer capable of helping my friend deal with her emotions. She is in shock. I can see signs of disbelief and depression. Fear has taken over her life and mine too.

Now I am realizing more and more that God has total control of our lives. But, He has given us free will and allows us to have choices. If we choose to believe in Him and believe His promises we will find that there is light at the end of the tunnel. It is at the end of every cancer diagnosis. THE LIGHT WILL SHINE FOR US. The same grace that brought us through our past is now promising us our future.

When we are confronted with challenges such as chemotherapy, radiation therapy and surgery, God comes to us with His promises. "I will never give you more than you can bear." "I will cause all things to work together for good." "Cast your burden upon the Lord and He will sustain you." "Call upon Him in the day of trouble and He will rescue you and you will honor Him."

Now I feel equipped. I can repeat God's promises to my friend and encourage her to visit that old Rugged Cross. There we will learn other steps necessary for our restoration.

While holding hands we skipped our way to the Cross as we sing that beautiful song written by Reverend George Bennard, "The Old Rugged Cross."

On a hill far away stood an old Rugged Cross.
The emblem of suffering and shame.
And I love that old Cross where the dearest and best for

A world of lost sinners was slain.
So I cherish the old Rugged Cross till my trophies at last
I lay down.
I will cling to the old Rugged Cross
And exchange it some day for a crown.

Oh that old Rugged Cross so despised by the world has a
Wondrous attraction for me.
For the dear Lamb of God left His glory above to bear it
To dark Calvary.

To the old Rugged Cross I will ever be true.
It's shame and reproach gladly bear.
Then He'll call me some day to my home far away where
His Glory forever I'll share.

I will cling to the old Rugged Cross and exchange it some
Day for a crown.

When God our Father wanted His son to become human, His son said, "Yes I will become man in order to restore creation in order to forgive their sins that they might have life."

When the Father wanted His son to eat nothing and be tempted by the Devil in the wilderness for forty days His son said "yes."

He never refused from doing what His Father wanted Him to do.

The cross was the ultimate "yes" spoken by Jesus to His Father. He said yes to his role as Savior of the whole world. He trusted His Father's plan and said, "Yes, I will lay down my life; I will make their sins mine; I will suffer the punishment they deserve; I will endure death for them that they might have life, eternal life."

God has been working throughout history to draw humanity back to Himself. From Genesis to Revelation we have one long story.

A story about how God loves us, even though we are disobedient, even though we deserve punishment. God is at work and shows us that there is a real problem. He tried to tell us how deep the breach is and just how far we are from what we should be. That is why He sent His son to save mankind.

First Peter 3:18, tells us, "For Christ also once suffered for sins, the just for the unjust that He might bring us to God; being put to death in the flesh, but quickened by the Spirit."

Jesus paid the price for our sins. He obtained pardon and forgiveness for all sinners. We are washed clean and made acceptable to God. God now offers us the hand of friendship and fellowship through His son. Jesus is our mediator for this new relationship. Now we can enjoy the status of being called the beloved children of God.

In respect to the cross, David Watson said:

> *"It is a picture of violence, yet the key to peace.*
> *It is a picture of suffering, yet the key to healing.*
> *It is a picture of death, yet the key to life.*
> *It is a picture of utter weakness, yet the key to power.*
> *It is a picture of capital punishment, yet the key to*
> *   Mercy and Forgiveness.*
> *It is a picture of vicious hatred, yet the key to love.*
> *It is a picture of supreme shame, yet the Christian's*
> *   supreme Boast."*

The cross reveals the nature of love. The cross shows us how much God loves us. The cross shows us an example of the love that we should emulate.

The cross conveys the power of a new life. Romans 6:6 "Our old way was nailed to the cross with Christ."

The cross brings healing and wholeness. One Peter 2:24. Because of the cross we can be healed and restored to wholeness-physically, mentally and spiritually.

As we made our way back from the cross, I realized that something was missing-my constant companion-my old self. Its absence felt odd and somewhat uncomfortable. For the past years it defined for me what was normal, but now it is no longer with me. My long mouth, my sad looking face are no longer a part of my identity. That old self is nailed to the cross.

I shared my experience with my friend and she said that she feels the same way too-her old self is left behind.

6

Experience His Presence

(Through Prayer, Praise And Pampering)

One way in which we can experience God's presence is to communicate with Him. And He invites us to do so.

Have you ever considered the nature of His gift. A gift granted by the Almighty Himself. We don't have to make an appointment to get His attention; We don't have to use our cell phones to reach Him. Instead, we are invited to call on Him at any moment, day or night.

We can pray standing up or sitting down. We can pray with our eyes open or closed. We can shout or we can be silent. What a privilege.

Our Lord describes Himself as a father. "As a father has compassion on his children, so the Lord has compassion on those who fear Him." Luke 11:13. He is also likened to a mother. "As a mother comforts her child so will I comfort you." Isaiah 66:13.

Pray He hears the faintest cry of the sick. The groan that seeps out in the night. The shrill scream of an anguished soul.

Pray the Bible gives us direction on how to do so. Luke 18:10-14.

Two men went up into the temple to pray. One a Pharisee and the other a Publican.

The Pharisee stood and prayed thus with himself, "God I thank thee that I am not as other men are, extortionists, unjust, adulterers or even as this Publican. I fast twice in the week, I give tithes of all that I possess.

And the Publican, standing afar off would not lift up so much as his eyes unto Heaven, but smote upon his breast saying, "God be merciful to me a sinner."

"I tell you this man went down to his house justified rather than the other. For everyone that exalteth himself shall be abashed and he that humbleth himself shall be exalted."

Further instructions were given by Jesus Himself. After this manner, therefore, pray he.

> *"Our Father which art in Heaven. Hallowed be Thy name. Thy Kingdom come. They will be done. On earth as it is in Heaven. Give us this day our daily bread. And forgive us our debts as we forgive our debtors. And lead us not into temptation, but deliver us from evil for thine is the kingdom and the power and the glory, forever. Amen.*

Matthew 6:9-13

Prayer is an essential tool for healing. God is the healer. He wants to heal those who are sick and hurting, but we have to give Him the opportunity to do so. Jesus has already paid the price for our healing. "He was bruised for our iniquities, the chastisement for our peace was upon Him and by His stripes we are healed. Isaiah 55:4-5.

James the apostle tells us that if anyone among us is afflicted we should pray for him, and if anyone is merry he should sing psalms.

James 5:14-16 states, "Is any sick among you? Let him call for the elders of the church and let them pray over him; anointing him with oil in the name of the Lord.

And the prayer of the faithful shall save the sick and the Lord shall raise him up and if he has committed sins they shall be forgiven him.

Confess your faults one to another and pray one for another that he may be healed. The effectual fervent prayer of a righteous man avails much."

Therefore, I say unto you what things so ever you desire when you pray believe that you receive them.

And when you stand praying, forgive if you have ought against any that your Father also which is in Heaven may forgive you your trespasses. But if you don't forgive neither will your Father which is in Heaven forgive your trespasses. Mark 11:24-26

Another way we can experience God's presence is to praise Him.

The Psalmist writes, "Enter into His gates with thanksgiving and into His courts with praise. Be thankful unto Him and bless His name. Psalms 100:4.

In order to praise God we must believe in Him. It is the kind of believing that releases the fountain of living water. The water we can share with others who are thirsty. It is the kind of believing that when tragedy strikes He will not let you fall. It is the kind of believing that when God touches your body there will not be a trace of cancer cells. It is the kind of believing that when God intervenes, not even your doctor can explain the process.

I, therefore, challenge you to become a person of praise and you will experience the release of the love and power of God.

The Bible tells us that God inhabits in the praise of His people.

Psalms 22:3. In other words, God dwells in an atmosphere of praise.

Praise is an expression of faith and a declaration of victory. It declares that we believe that God is in control of the outcome of all our challenges. We also know that all things work together for good to them that love God, to them who are called according to His purpose. Romans 8:28.

Praise means to commend, to applaud or magnify. It is an expression of worship.

It magnifies our awareness of our spiritual union with the most high God.

It is an expression of humility as we center our attention upon the Lord with heartfelt expression of love, adoration and thanksgiving.

Praise is a vehicle of faith which brings us into the presence and power of God.

"Praise ye the Lord for it is good to sing praises unto our God. Psalms 147:1.

"Rejoice in the Lord always and again I say rejoice. Let your moderation be known unto all men. The Lord is at hand.

Be careful for nothing; but in everything by prayer and supplication with thanksgiving let your requests be made known unto God.

And the peace of God which passeth all understanding shall keep your hearts and minds through Christ Jesus." Phillipians 4:4-8.

I give God the glory and praise for working a miracle in my life. Like David, I will sing unto the Lord as long as I live. I will sing praise to my God while I have my being. Psalms 104:33.

I am reminded of a patient who was sitting in a wheelchair with both hands resting on her head.

"What's wrong?" I asked. With a sad face, she looked up at me and said, "Here I am hungry and lonely and my husband could not spend another minute with me. He had to run home to pet the dogs."

The need for physical closeness and pampering seem to become most apparent when sickness strikes, yet it seems that some of us are fearful of giving it. These are simple human acts. A pat on the back, a hug-this represents common physical expression of affection and understanding. How wonderful it would be to learn the process from an awkward embrace to one that ended with a true expression of "I love you." This type of embrace heals. It has the power to seep deep into the aching heart and soothe the soul.

Pampering. This is another way we can experience God's presence. Galatians 5:13 instructs us to serve one another. When we become God's hands serving others through love, when we make ourselves available to assist the wounded, when we create an environment of warmth and consideration for those who are struggling with cancer or any other disease we are inviting God's presence. Most of us are aware of the needs of the sick. In many cases they are not asking for much. If we truly care we should be willing to relinquish a part of ourselves for their joy. We should be willing to pamper them every step of the way.

Pampering means speaking comfortably and carefully to the wounded at all times. Encourage them to remain positive. Encouragement yields results all the time.

It is the power of the spoken word that moves us. It will move us forward or it will demolish us.

Because of this dreaded disease people's dreams are shattered and relationships broken. Most often it is because of the tongue. Most of us have been victims of thoughtless words and we too suffer the consequences. Before we speak we should weigh the affects of our words.

It is amazing to think that something as small as your tongue can destroy relationships and ruin opportunities. It is small, quick and deadly. The people who really love you, your bedridden mates who want to be with you, are most likely the ones to become wounded by your words.

Your real enemies will never be affected by what you say because they pay you nor your words any attention.

The Bible teaches us that the power of life and death is in the tongue. Proverbs 18:21.

It also tells us that the words of a tale bearer are as wounds and they go down into the innermost parts of the belly. Proverbs 18:8. Please don't hurt the wounded or the depressed with a tongue that is out of control.

There are times when you can speak without opening your

mouth. Your hands and eyes can often send louder and clearer messages if they are used the right way.

You have been given a swift tongue, so use it to speak peace to the storms of life and speak blessings and petition Heaven on behalf of your loved ones.

My sister, who was involved in a terrible car accident, slipped into a coma. Her heart stopped beating and was resuscitated four times. Four different times. The doctors gave up all hope, but her family never did.

Relatives and friends prayed for her. It was not only the strong prayers that pulled her through, it was the familiar voices of her sisters that made her climb out of the arms of death.

When you speak you can call the sick from a state of depression or despair. You can speak healing and blessings in their ears. Your tongue has the power. For God's sake use it for good.

I am reminded of my mother, such a beautiful woman, who has the ingredients of love and family orientation. She transformed the house my father built into a home. She is a woman of great strength and power and an abundance of class which she demonstrates. With her well tailored dress draped with an apron, she would walk throughout the house making sure everything was in its place. Although she had helpers, she always put the finishing touches on our meals. The smell of fried dumplings, plantains, ackee, salt fish, roast beef, brown stew, chicken, the sounds of laughter and the touch of affection were everyday occurrences. There was no television screen in the early days, but family games were in abundance.

As I am writing, my mother is getting dressed for church with her hat, stockings and pocketbook to match her pumps. The dress is something to behold. She is not leaving for church without encouraging everyone who is present to find a church to go to. A fascinating woman she is. If you are sick, expect to be pampered royally. Hot milk and ginger tea or fever grass tea will be served to you on a tray. The bizzy tea will follow if there is any indication that allergic reaction is present. Her very touch warms the core of your soul. That is pampering.

Pamper yourself. "The first affair that we must consummate successfully is the love affair with ourselves," says Nathaniel Branden in his book The Psychology of Romantic Love. "Only then are we ready for other love relationships."

Light a candle, set a table for one and dream. Dreams enrich the future with possibilities. Dream of peace, pleasure and joy and places to visit.

There is joy in planning even if the dream is not realized. DREAM.

Pamper yourself. There are some songs that will bring comfort to your soul. The first one was written in 1916 by C. Albert Tindley. Sing it in the morning, sing it at noon. Just sing it.

"Leave it there, leave it there.

Take your burden to the Lord and leave it there.

If you trust and never doubt He will surely bring you out.

Take your burden to the Lord and leave it there."

When you get up in the mornings just whisper these words written by George Stebbins in 1935.

"Have thine own way Lord. Have thine own way. Thou are the potter. I am the clay. Mold me and make me after Thy will. While I am waiting, yielded and still."

At bedtime just hum this cleansing prayer, written by Edwin Orr.

"Search me God and know my heart today. Try me, O Savior, know my thoughts I pray. See if there be some wicked way in me. Cleanse me from every sin and set me free."

Pamper yourself. It is time to take a happy bath. A bath that will remind you of your own healing experiences and bring forth your great testaments.

Pamper yourself upon waking in the mornings. Take some deep cleansing breaths. Inhale through your nose and exhale through your mouth. Take a walk in the garden. Listen and enjoy the chirping sounds of the birds. Look around at the beautiful trees and flowers. Look up at the sky with the interesting cloud formation. Listen to music. Music brings a sense of well-being to us and seems to distract us from the weary road we are traveling.

Enjoy your own company. Value your existence and experience God's presence. Pamper yourself. It is through pampering that you find comfort and peace.

Pray to your Creator. Raise your hands and smile at a God you cannot see. Embrace your God through prayer, praise and pampering.

Now just sit back, relax and trust God. The universe is full of delightful surprises if we will just allow it to tell its own story and provide direction without interference.

7

Jesus Our Miracle Worker

Receive thy sight. Your faith hath saved thee.

Luke 18:42

In order to understand and appreciate the miracles of Jesus, one first has to understand what a miracle is and then consider why Jesus would make them such an integral part of His ministry.

In general terms, miracles may be defined as supernatural manifestations of divine power.

The miracles of Jesus not only established His identity, but also make His promises credible. "I will never leave you nor forsake you. Call upon me in the day of trouble and I will rescue you and you will honor Me. Cast your burden upon Me and I will sustain you."

Jesus' primary reason for coming into the world was not to perform miracles. "His goal was to seek and to save that which was lost." Luke 10:10.

The works He performed were a means to that end. His miraculous works caused many people to follow Him in order to be healed, but Jesus wanted them to follow Him for His message of salvation.

When Jesus worked wonders among the people and healing

them of their afflictions and diseases, He was showing them the deliverance they could have from their greatest affliction - sin.

His miracles showed that He has the power to forgive sin and that forgiveness of sin was of greater concern to Him than physical healing.

To the paralytic He said, "Your sins are forgiven thee. Arise and walk."

The ability of Jesus to speak and calm the wind and the sea had a profound effect upon those in the boat with Him.

Even though His disciples had seen Him perform miracles previous to this, they were still awed by the open demonstration of the power of God before them.

When he was awakened by the voice of His disciples, "He rebuked the wind and the sea and commanded them to be still."

"Then Jesus went about all the cities and villages, teaching in their synagogues, preaching the gospel of the Kingdom and healing every sickness and every disease among the people. But, when He saw the multitudes He was moved with compassion for them because they were weary and scattered like sheep having no shepherd." Then He said to His disciples, "The harvest truly is plentiful, but the laborers are few. Therefore, pray the Lord of the harvest to send out laborers into His harvest." Matthew 9:35-38.

As we examine this passage, let us ask the Holy Spirit to teach us the ways that Jesus Himself showed compassion to the needy. Let us ask the Holy Spirit to make us more like our Savior who shows great compassion towards us.

Verse 35 reads, "Jesus went about all the cities and villages." This is an example for us. We should not wait for the sick to come to us. We should go to them and tell them about the healing power of Jesus. We should write letters to them, send cards. Don't wait until they make the first move. Go to them, sit with them.

The next thing Jesus did was to serve them. He taught them, He preached to them, He told them the good news of the Kingdom and urged them to respond to it.

Jesus met the physical, spiritual and emotional needs of those he went to. He healed every sickness and disease among the people.

Nicodemus, the ruler of the Jews, who came to Him by night, knew that Jesus had come from God because of the work he had seen Jesus do. He said, "Rabbi, we know that you are a teacher come from God; for no one can do these signs that you do unless God is with him. John 3:2.

Why did Jesus perform miracles? Jesus answered this question Himself. When in prison, John the Baptist sent some of His disciples to Jesus to see if He was the one to come. (Matthew 11:3) Jesus told them to inform John of what He had done. "The blind receive sight, the lame walk, those who have leprosy are cured, the deaf hear, the dead are raised and the good news preached to the poor. (Matthew 11:5) With these words, Jesus declared that His miracles were the fulfillment of the promises of the Messiah's Kingdom as foretold by Isaiah. (Isaiah 24: 18-19; 35: 5-6; 61: 1) Jesus' miracles were signs of the presence of the Kingdom of God. (Matthew 12:29)

John 14: 12-14 reads, "He who believes in me, the works that I do, he will do also and greater works than these he will do; because I go to my Father and whatever you ask in My name that I will do, that the Father may be glorified in the Son. If you ask anything in My name I will do it."

Jesus, our miracle worker, used different healing resources when He performed some of the miracles. He healed a blind man by putting mud on his eyes.

"He spat on the ground and made clay from the spittle and anointed the eyes of the blind man and said, "Go wash in the pool of Siloam." John 9: 6-7.

And God wrought special miracles by the hand of Paul. So that from His body were brought unto the sick handkerchiefs or aprons and the diseases departed from them. Acts 19:11.

And there sat a certain man at Haystra, impotent in his feet being a cripple from his mother's womb who never had walked.

The same heard Paul speak who steadfastly beholding him perceiving that he had faith to be healed, said with a loud voice, "Stand upright on thy feet. And he leaped and walked." Acts 14: 8-10.

Jesus healed Bartimaeus. What wilt thou that I shall do unto thee and he said Lord that I may receive my sight. And Jesus said unto him, "Receive thy sight. Thy faith hath saved thee." And immediately he received his sight. Luke 18: 41-43.

I can hear that sweet soft voice repeating those words. "Lorna, thy faith hath saved thee."

One of my doctors told me that the amount of chemo and radiation that I received could not cure my disease.

Did Jesus use the Sour Sop tree as His resource to restore my health?

My friend God is real. He is awesome.

When I was sitting in the surgeon's office I felt nervous. I took some deep breaths, inhaling through my nostrils and exhaling through my mouth and hoped to remain calm.

"Hi, Mrs. Richardson. How are you today?" the surgeon asked. "Oh, I feel great, thank you." I replied. "What effects did the chemo have on your body?" "Oh, it was like a tonic." I replied. "My hair grew. I gained weight. My lab results are very good. I had no nausea or vomiting." "What about your radiation therapy?" he asked. "I had six delightful weeks of therapy", I replied.

After six weeks, the staff presented me with a certificate certifying that I was an outstanding patient, always pleasant and jovial, signed by the MD and other members of the radiation team. It made my day.

"And now it is time to have the tumor removed. The type of surgery that is scheduled depends on the location of the tumor. If the tumor is located at the lower end of the colon we will do an abdominal peritoneal resection with a permanent colostomy. "Do you mind if I do a rectal examination on you?" "Not at all" I replied.

The rectal examination was done. There was silence. What is my surgeon thinking? Is he trying to put his thoughts together? Is he wondering how best he could discuss the findings? He knows how delicate life is and how fragile the heart and mind can be if they are not handled with care.

"Did you feel the tumor?", I asked. "No, did the emergency room doctor feel it?, he asked. "Yes, she did", I replied.

There was still silence. My husband was invited in the examining room. The computer was turned on the he was shown the repeated CAT Scan results. I became curious. "Doctor, could you show me the tumor?" Now there were three pairs of eyes chasing after the tumor. We looked to the north and to the south, to the east and to the west. The doctor then looked at both of us and said, "I cannot see the tumor." The next question from me was "Can you identify the location?" "No, I can't, but I will check with the doctor who first diagnosed you." was his reply. "Doctor, I saw the CAT Scan report and it did not identify any malignant tumor." "Doctor, I am healed. God touched me and blew the tumor away without leaving a trace. There are no signs or symptoms of the disease. God touched me and made me whole. The tumor cannot be seen, cannot be felt, nor can the location be identified."

God heard my cry and moved into action. He stood between the surgeon and myself and said, "How can you remove a tumor you cannot see? How can you remove a tumor without knowing its location? How can you remove a tumor you cannot feel?"

The surgeon sat on the stool, looked me in the eyes and said, "Lorna, tell me something about yourself." I quickly replied, "I am a Christian and I believe God's word. I am a member of the Church of God of Prophecy and I am a Registered Nurse."

There was silence.

God reached down and tenderly removed me from my surgeon's grip.

The surgeon looked at me, then said, "Come back and see me in six months."

Why does God do all this? Why respond to His child's cry with such power and force?

God has to demonstrate His power to show us who is in control and why it is necessary to switch our focus from our earthly physician to our heavenly one. He has to demonstrate His power to show that He is Omnipotent and He is our Creator.

He has to demonstrate His power to show that before Him there was no other God. Neither shall there be after Him. Isaiah 43:10.

But, why did he do it for me. Because I believe His word and trust Him.

"Call upon me in the day of trouble and I will rescue you." Thus saith the Lord.

How could I not love a God who picked, bagged and sent me my healing medication.

How could I not tremble in the presence of my God knowing that He stooped down and with His scalpel cleansed and removed that monster.

How could I not love and appreciate a God who assumed the task of an attorney and defended me. A God who stood between my surgeon and myself.

How can you not love a God who required no fees and wins the case for His glory and for my good.

Why shouldn't I wash His feet with my tears and kiss His nail scarred hands.

Why shouldn't I?

I am also reminded of my mother who loves the Lord. A God-fearing lady who is ninety-six years old. Alert, strong, healthy and who ambulates independently. Never had surgery. No major illness. She always told us that the cure for diseases can be found in our garden. For example, if she had chest pain she would make tea from the leaf that resembles the heart. For a cold it would be tea from the "leaf of life" plant. This plant resembles the lung. For diabetes it is a leaf that resembles the pancreas. For urinary problems it is a leaf that resembles the kidney.

When I told her my dream, she said "I am not surprised because 'sour sop' has a crusty skin and reminds me of cancer."

Lately, I am receiving calls from relatives and friends telling me of their healing experiences which they attributed to God and the sour sop tree.

I know if it were not for the grace of God, I would be wearing a colostomy bag today. Probably, a permanent one. This would be a little more than I could bear at this time in my life. But, I know that one of God's promises is that He will not give us more than we can bear and I prove Him over and over again.

God saw how weak and helpless I had become so he whispered in my ears, "My grace is sufficient for thee. For my strength is made perfect in weakness." 2 Corinthians 12: 9. Our weakness is the environment in which God's power thrives.

I know my weakness set the stage for His presence in the doctor's office.

Powerlessness can scare us, but it is through our weakness, our hardships, our difficulties God works and shows His greatness.

All we have to do is trust Him. He is our Creator. He is our father, our mother. "As a shepherd carried his lamb I have carried you close to my heart saith the Lord." Isaiah 40:11. "I will never leave thee nor forskake thee." How comforting are these words.

God is my Creator, my father, my mother. He knows what is best for me. If my life is prolonged for a day, a week, a month, a year, 10 years, 20 years, I will give Him all the praise and glory as long as I live.

8

Restoration

Weeping may endure for a night but joy cometh in the morning.

Psalm 30. 5

God makes beauty out of our damaged and broken lives. He is a restorer, a redeemer. The Bible tells us in Isaiah 51: 3, "For the Lord shall comfort Zion. He will comfort all her waste places and He will make her wilderness like Eden and her desert like the Garden of the Lord. Joy and gladness shall be found therein. Thanksgiving and the voice of melody."

When we are experiencing our challenging moments, feeling weak, useless and inadequate, restoration looks completely out of reach. We know that it is what we need, but we think it is impossible to obtain. But, it is not so. God loves us just the way we are. He loves us unconditionally. He will restore us. That is His promise to us.

God has a purpose for our lives. He has a plan for us. He has designated a life for us designed for Kingdom work for His glory and for our good.

God is saying to each of us, "Where you place your foot, the ground is yours; where you walk, it is yours. You are victorious wherever you go if you are with Me and in Me." Joshua 1: 3.

This is the promise God gave to Joshua many years ago and today He is giving us the same promise. In addition, He is commanding us to "be strong and of good courage, be not afraid neither be thou dismayed. For the Lord Thy God is with thee wither soever thou goest." Joshua 1:9.

The God we must learn to know is God the Father, maker of Heaven and earth, the only wise God, our Savior. He is the one who brings out the starry hosts by number and calls them all by name through the greatness of His power.

We can never appreciate our Savior until we recognize Him as our creator and sovereign God.

Fear Him and give Him all the glory. The Bible says the fear of the Lord is the beginning of wisdom. Psalm 111:10.

God must become the focal point of our lives as we daily strive to love Him with all our hearts, our souls and our minds. If we take the time to ask God for the answers that we seek, and if we are still and silent long enough, God will speak to us in whatever way needed so that we will hear Him clearly.

The Bible teaches, "Be still and know that I am God." Psalm 46: 10. "Stand in awe and sin not. Commune with your own heart upon your bed and be still." Psalm 4:4.

We all have a special role to play in this life. We are all sinners saved by His grace. We make mistakes, we sin, we fail, but Jesus is very comfortable working with broken people. There are many examples throughout the Holy Scriptures where God restored and used broken people. For example, Moses, Paul, Peter. When we experience brokenness we do not have to hide behind our mask. God wants to restore us and use us for His glory. All we have to do is to open our hearts and ask the Holy Spirit to guide us once again. God has plans for us. Plans to give us a future and a hope.

The Book of Job tells the story of a man who lost everything; his wealth, his family and his health and wrestles with the question why. And guess what? "The Lord blessed the latter end of Job more than the beginning." Job 42:12.

Jeremiah 30: 17 states, "For I will restore health unto thee and I will heal thee of thy wounds saith the Lord."

Sometimes God restores us, but leaves the scars. These scars will remind us of the pain we once endured. They also remind us of His ability and His love. Our scars are also living testimony. Other people need to know what God has done for us.

God wants to use our lives, our stories, our dreams and scars for His glory and our good.

Let us take a quick look at the apostle Peter's restoration.

When Jesus asked His disciples, "Who do men think I am?" the answer was, "John the Baptist, Elias and others." Then Jesus asked, "But, whom say ye that I am?" Matthew 16:15. Simon Peter answered, "Thou art the Christ, the Son the living God." Peter declared his love for Jesus. Peter also defended Jesus by cutting off the high priest's servant's ear with a sword. Jesus forgave Peter and healed the ear.

Peter who has been with Jesus for so long, who knows who Jesus was, who loved Him, who gave up everything to follow Him; denied Jesus, not once, but three times. Peter swore, saying he did not know that man. Can you imagine how Peter felt at the end of the day. No doubt he was loosing his mind. he probably prayed for an opportunity to tell Jesus how sorry, how devastated, how broken he was.

After the Resurrection, Jesus appears unto Peter and asks, "Simon, son of Jonas, lovest thou Me more than thee?" Peter's reply was, "Yea Lord, thou knowest that I love Thee."

Jesus repeated the same question three times and told Peter three times to feed His lambs. John 21:15.

This experience helped Peter to become aware of his limitations and his brokenness.

Peter sinned, failed and made mistakes. Jesus restored him and took him beyond where he was.

Peter was the first to declare the gospel to the Gentiles. He was the first to preach the gospel publicly.

Matthew 16:18. "And I say unto thee that thou art Peter and

upon this rock I will build My church and the gates of Hell shall not prevail against it."

This is truly restoration. Jesus met Peter where he was and pushed him forward.

Jesus wants to do the same for you, and He will if you allow Him to.

Sometimes God tries to communicate with us by sending signs and symbols. Job 33:14 states, "he hath spoken once yea twice, yet man perceiveth it not."

God also visits us and sends messages through dreams. "The prophet that has a dream, let him tell a dream. And he that hath my word, let him speak it faithfully." Jeremiah 23: 28.

I am compelled to speak His word faithfully because I had a dream and I also recognize His sings and symbols. The Sour Sop Tree.

God wants to restore you. The Sour Sop Tree might be His resource. Who knows? He wants to meet you where you are and birth you with a new beginning. He wants your broken pieces, your shattered hopes and dreams, your broken relationships, your malignant tumors.

God knows how pregnant you are with fear and uncertainty.

His plan is to restore you. He knows that you are in pain. He knows how badly burnt you are from radiation therapy. He knows you lost weight, you look twice your age with no hair on your head. But, don't give up. Don't give in.

The pain you are having now could be a contraction signaling the beginning of the birthing process.

You are approaching the end of the tunnel. Get ready for your delivery. You may want to invite some of your relatives and friends in the room with you to witness your restoration.

The pain is getting worse. The contractions are more frequent. This is not the time to give up. Hold onto your mate. Hold onto your nurse. Grab the bars of the bed and PUSH! PUSH! PUSH! Men enjoy some deep breaths, delivery is just around the corner for you too.

The next PUSH might be the one that will rid the body of the last cancer cell or release the emotions you have suppressed over the years or the grip you have on your past wounds. PUSH! PUSH! PUSH! WOW, WOW, what a relief, what a wonderful and glorious feeling. Now there is light.

This is the release of God's love and power.

This is the reward for leaving your sins at the foot of the cross.

This is the reward for letting go of anger and blame.

This is the reward for holding onto God during that painful divorce.

This is the reward for hiding your kids in the closet so that they won't witness the abuse and crime scenes.

This is the reward for turning the next cheek.

This is the reward for not pulling the trigger.

This is the reward for those who have been pulled to the breaking point.

You can never know how free you are, how healthy you have become until you understand how pregnant you once were with broken pieces, fear and uncertainly. Some of us would not be as focused today if it were not for our struggle and finally our delivery.

God bless you all.

9

Devotion Time

The following verses were selected from the Holy Scriptures. They can be used during devotion or as a starting point for praising God.

I pray that as we read together His words, our load will be lighter and we will become happier knowing that God indeed cares for us and loves us with an everlasting love.

These verses will empower us through the best and worst of times.

Designed to be read daily repeating the schedule every 30-31 days.

Let's sing as we start our daily devotion.

Turn your eyes upon Jesus, look full in His wonderful face and the things of earth will grow strangely dim in the light of His glory and grace.

This is a special prayer.

I pray it will bless you the way it blessed me.

HEAVENLY FATHER,

I call on You right now in a special way. It is through Your power that I was created. Every breath I take, every morning I wake, every moment of every hour, I live under Your power.

Father, I ask You now to touch me with that same power. For if You created me from nothing, You can certainly recreate me. Fill me with the healing power of Your Spirit. Cast out anything that should not be in me. Mend what is broken. Root out any unproductive cell. Open any blocked arteries or veins and rebuild any damaged areas. Remove all inflammation and cleanse any infection.

Let the warmth of Your healing love pass through my body to make new any unhealthy area so that my body will function the way You created it to function.

And Father, restore me to full health in mind and body so that I may serve You the rest of my life.

I ask this through Christ our Lord.

Amen.

DAY 1

<u>God Predetermines the Events of Life</u>

To every thing there is a season and a time
To every purpose under the heavens.

Ecclesiastes 3.1

A time to be born and a time to die, a time to plant and a
time to pluck up that which is planted.

Ecclesiastes 3.2

A time to get and a time to lose. A time to keep and a
time to cast away.

Ecclesiastes e.6

DAY 2

God Predetermines the Condition of Life

Every man shall eat and drink and enjoy the good of all
his labor.
It is the gift of God.

Ecclesiasts 3.13

I know that whatsoever God doeth it shall be forever;
nothing can be put to it nor anything taken from it
and God doeth it.
That man should fear before Him.

Ecclesiastes 3.14

Eye hath not seen nor ear heard. Neither have entered
into the heart of man the things which God hath
prepared for them that love Him.

1 Corinthians 2.9

DAY 3

God's Promises

Surely blessing I will bless thee and multiplying I will multiply thee.

Hebrews 6.14

Fear thou not for I am with thee, be not dismayed for I am they God.
I will strengthen thee, yea I will help thee, yea I will uphold thee with
The right hand of my righteousness.

Isaiah 41.10

I will never leave thee nor forsake thee.

Hebrews 13.5

If you abide in me and my words abide in you, ask whatever you wish
And it will be done for you.

John 15.7

Cast they burden upon the Lord and He shall sustain thee. He shall never suffer the righteous to be moved.

Psalm 56.13

DAY 4

God Will Provide For You

Take no thought for your life what ye shall drink nor yet
for your body what ye shall put on. Is not the life
more than meat and the boy more than raiment?
Behold the fowls of the air for they sow not neither
do they reap nor gather into barns. Yet your
Heavenly Father feedeth them. Are you not
much better than they?

Matthew 6.25–26

DAY 5

<u>God's Grace</u>

The Lord is my shepherd; I shall not want. He maketh
  me to lie down in green pastures; He leadeth me
  beside the still waters.
He restoreth my soul; He leadeth me in the path of
  righteousness for his name's sake.
Yea, though I walk through the valley of the shadow of
  death I will fear no evil; for thou art with me; thy
  rod and they staff they comfort me.
Thou prepares a table before me in the presence of mine
  enemies.
Thou anointed my head with oil, my cup runneth over.
Surely goodness and mercy shall follow me all the days
  of my life and
I will dwell in the house of the Lord forever.

Psalm 23.1-6

DAY 6

<u>Praise</u>

And their sins and iniquities will I remember no more.

Hebrews 10.17

Praise the Lord for His mercy endureth forever.

2 Chronicles 20.21

Sing praises to the Lord which dwelleth in Zion.
Declare among the people His doings.

Psalm 9.16

The Lord is my strength and my shield; my heart trusted
in Him and I am helped. Therefore, my heart
greatly rejoyceth and with my song
Will I praise Him.

Psalm 28.7

I will sing unto the Lord, because He hath dealt
bountifully with me.

Psalm 13.6

DAY 7

How much more can I take?

Change focus from pain to His promises.
A very pleasant help in trouble.

Psalm 46.1

The Lord is my helper and I will not fear what man shall do unto me.

Hebrews 13.6

I will seek that which was lost and bring again that which was driven away and will bind up that which was broken and will strengthen that which was sick.

Ezekiel 34.16

And we know that all things work together for good to them that love God, to them who are called according to His purpose.

Romans 8.28

DAY 8

Jesus paid the price for our healing

For I will restore health unto thee and I will heal thee of thy wounds.

Jeremiah 30.17

God is a restorer and a redeemer.

Isaiah 51.3

He was bruised for our iniquities. The chastisement for our peace was upon Him and by His stripes we are healed.

Isaiah 55.4–5

DAY 9

God dwells in an atmosphere of Praise

God inhabits in the praise of His people.

Psalm 22.3

Enter into His gates with thanksgiving and into His courts with praise.
Be thankful unto Him and bless His name.

Psalm 100.4

I will sing praise to my God while I have my being.

Psalm 104.33

DAY 10

Don't Worry

"Peace I leave with you and peace I give unto you. Not as the world giveth give I unto you let not your heart be troubled neither let it be afraid.

John 14.27

Count it all joy when ye fall into diverse temptation. Knowing this that the trying of your faith worketh patience."

James 1-2&3

The secret things belong to the Lord our God.

Deutoronomy 29.29

DAY 11

<u>Do not be afraid</u>

Let not your heart be troubled neither let it be afraid.

John 14.27

There is no fear in love but perfect love casteth out fear.

As a shepherd carries his lamb I have carried you close to my heart. Sayeth the Lord.

Isaiah 40.11

Fear thou not for I am with thee. Be not dismayed for I am thy God. I will strengthen thee. Yea I will uphold thee with the right hand of my righteousness.

Isaiah 41.10

DAY 12

Don't Be Discouraged

And let us not be weary in well doing. For in due season we shall reap if we faint not.

Galatians 6.9

Cast no away therefore your confidence which has great Recompense of reward.

Hebrews 10.35

Come unto me all ye that labour and are heavily laden and I will give you rest.

Matthew 11.28

DAY 13

__Let God be God__

For my thoughts are not your thoughts.
Neither are your ways my ways declares the Lord.

Isaiah 55.89

Lean not on your own understanding.

Proverbs 3.5

The secret things belong to the Lord our God.

Deuteronomy 29.29

DAY 14

You have a special role to play

If you seek Him you will find Him.

Deuteronomy 4.29

Rejoice in as much as ye are partakers of Christ
suffering that when His glory shall be revealed ye
may be glad also with exceeding joy.

1st Peter 4.12–13

Happy is the man who God correcteth;
Therefore despise not thou the chastening of the
Almighty.

Job 5.17

And let us not be weary in well doing;
For in due season we shall reap if we faint not.

Galatians 6.9

DAY 15

How to Inherit Eternal Life

Thou shalt love the Lord thy God with all they heart
an with all thy soul and with all they strength and
with all they mind and they neighbour as thyself.
And He said unto him, thou hast answered right.
This do and thou shalt live.

Deuteronomy 6.5

Blessed are the pure in heart for they shall see God.

Matthew 5.8

Love your enemies bless them that curse you. Do good
to them that hate you and pray for them which
despitefully use you and persecute you.

Matthew 5.44

DAY 16

<u>You do the possible and let God do the impossible</u>

My grace is sufficient for you for My power is made perfect in weakness.

2d Corinthians 12.9

I will go before thee and make the crooked places straight. I will break in pieces the gates of brass and cut in sunder the bards of iron.

Isaiah 45.2

With god all things are possible.

Matthew 19.26

DAY 17

Prayer for Guidance

Show me they ways O Lord; Teach me Thy paths.
Lead me in Thy truth and tech me; for Thou art the
God of my salvation.
On Thee do I wait all the day.

Psalm 24.4-5

Teach me O Lord the way of my statutes and I will keep it
Unto the end.
Give me understanding and I shall keep Thy law. Yea I
Shall observe it with my whole heart.
Make me to go in the path of Thy commandments;
For therein do I delight.

Psalm 119.33-35

DAY 18

Comfort

*Let not your heart be troubled, ye believe in God believe
Also in me.*

John 14.1

*In my father's house are many mansions. If it were not so
I would have told you I go to prepare a place for you.
I will come again and receive you unto myself;
That where I am there ye may be also.*

John 14.1-3

*The Lord also will be a refuge for the oppressed;
A refuge in times of trouble.*

Psalm 9.9

*As one who his mother comforted,
So will I comfort you.*

Isaiah 66.13

*I have been young and now I am old; yet have I not
seen the righteous forsaken nor his seed begging
bread.*

Psalm 37.25

DAY 19

<u>Words to Guide you</u>

Except the Lord build the house, they labor in vain that built it; Except the Lord keep the city, the watchman waketh but in vain.

Psalm 127.1

I will instruct thee and teach thee in the way which thou shalt go. I will guide thee with mine eyes.

Psalm 32.8

Get all the advice you can and be wise the rest of your life.

Proverbs 19.20

Let love and faithfulness never leave you. Bind them around your neck. Write them on the table of your heart.

Proverbs 3.3

Let your light so shine before men, that they may see your good works and glorify your Father who is in Heaven.

Proverbs 20.20

Why beholdest thou the mote that is in they brother's eye, but Perceivist not the beam that is in your own eye.

Luke 6.41

DAY 20

Wait upon the Lord

Truly my soul waited upon God;
From Him cometh my salvation.

Psalms 62.1

My soul wait thou only upon God for my expectation is
from Him.

Psalms 62.5

Show me Thy ways O Lord. Teach me Thy path.
Lead me in Thy truth and teach me for Thou art the
God of my salvation.
On Thee do I wait all the day.

Psalms 25.4–5

DAY 21

God is not Mocked

Be not deceived. God is not mocked. For whatsoever a man saveth that shall he also reap.

Galatians 6.7

Behold we count them happy which endure. Ye have heard of the patience of Job and have seen the end of the Lord; and the Lord is very pitiful and of tender mercy.

James 5.1

DAY 22

For those who are mourning

Precious in the sight of the Lord is the death of His saints.

Psalm 116.15

Blessed are they who mourn for they will be comforted.

Matthew 5.4

Don't see death as a tragedy. See it as a triumph.
Paul put it this way. Oh death where is they sting;
Oh grave where is thy victory.

1st Corinthians 15.55

DAY 23

<u>Happy Days</u>

Forsake her not and she shall preserve thee;
Love her and she shall keep thee.

Proverbs 4.6

He that despiseth his neighbor sinneth; but he that hath
mercy on the poor happy is he.

Proverbs 14.21

The wife shall be as a fruitful vine by the sides of thine
houses;
Thy children like olive plants round about thy table.

Psalm 128.3

For thou shalt eat the laborer of thine hands; happy
shalt thou be and it shall be well with thee.

Psalm 128.2

DAY 24

When you feel lonely

I will never leave you. I will never forsake you.

Hebrew 13.5

When you pass through the waters I will be there with you.

Isaiah 43.2

I am with you always.

Matthew 28.26

DAY 25

Love

For as high as the heavens are above the earth
So great is His love for those who fear Him.

Psalm 103.11

The eyes of the Lord are on the righteous and the ears
are attentive to their prayers.

Peter 3.12

Love worketh no ill to his neighbor.
Therefore love is the fulfilling of the law.

Romans 12.10

DAY 26

Definition of Faith

Faith is the substance of things hoped for.
The evidence of things not seen.

Hebrews 11.1

Without Faith it is impossible to please God.
For he that cometh God must believe that He is and
that He is a reward of them that diligently seek
Him.

Hebrews 11.6

The prayer of Faith shall same the sick and the Lord
shall raise him up and if he have committed sins
they shall be forgiven him.

James 5.15

DAY 27

God is Worthy to be Praised

Great is the Lord and greatly to be praised;
And His greatness is unsearchable.

Psalm 145.3

The Lord is gracious and full of compassion, slow to
anger and of great mercy.

Psalm 145.8

The Lord is good to all and His tender mercies are over
all His works.

Psalm 145.9

DAY 28

God Heals the Brokenhearted

have mercy upon me O Lord for I am weak
O Lord heal me for my bones are vexed.

Psalm 6.2

And he shall be like a tree planted by the rivers of
water, that bringeth forth his fruit in his season.
His leaves shall not wither and whatsoever he
doeth shall prosper.

Psalm 1.3

God healeth the broken in heart and bindeth up their
wounds.

Psalm 147.3

DAY 29

Be Wise

Humble yourselves in the sight of the Lord and
He shall lift you up.

James 4.10

He that is slow to anger is better than the mighty and he
that ruleth his spirit than he that taketh a city.

Proverbs 16.32

For God speaketh once, yea twice, yet man perceiveth it
not.

Job 33.14

The fear of God is the beginning of wisdom and
knowledge of the Holy is understanding.

Proverbs 9.10

DAY 30

Woman thou art Loosed

*And when Jesus saw her He called her to Him and
said unto her woman thou art loosed from thine
infirmity.
And He laid His hands on her and immediately she
was made straight and glorified God.*

Luke 13.12–13

*Cast me not away from thy presence and take not thy
holy Spirit from me.*

Psalm 51.11

*Restore unto me the joy of thy salvation and uphold me
with thy free spirit.*

Psalm 51.12

DAY 31

The Dream

The prophet that has a dream let him tell a dream and he that
Hath my word let him speak faithfully.

Jeremiah 23.28

For God speaketh once, yea twice; yet man perceiveth it not.

Job 33.14

About The Author

Lorna D. Marshall-Richardson earned her Registered Nurse diploma from the University of The West Indies, Jamaica and her Batchelor of Science degree and a Master of Science degree in Health Care Management from Florida International University.

She is the author of *Don't You Ever Give Up-A Message for Teens and Young Adults* and also *It's Harvest Time.*

Along with her husband, they owned and operated a real estate business for many years.

They both have two children, Karlene and Gary and five grandchildren, Tia, Teddy, Lexcy, Lenae and Jada.

E-mail: Thecocktail2011@hotmail.com

www.ingramcontent.com/pod-product-compliance
Lightning Source LLC
Chambersburg PA
CBHW030358290526
45785CB00004B/1813